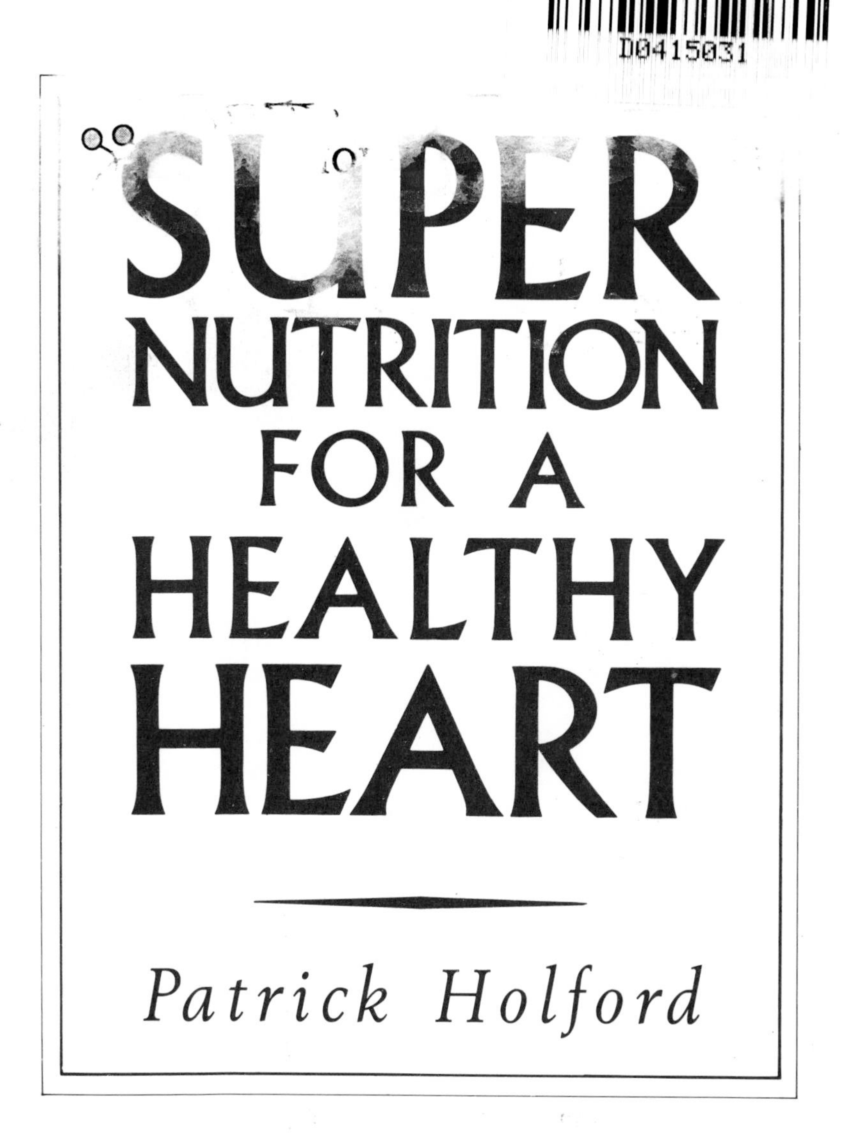

SUPER NUTRITION FOR A HEALTHY HEART

Patrick Holford

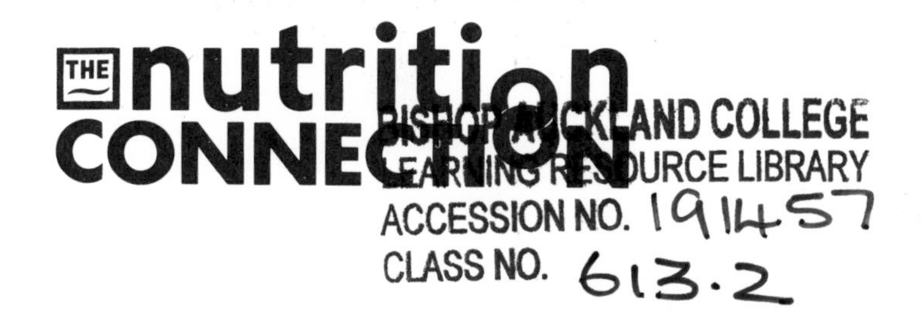

First published in 1989
by ION Press, a division of The Institute for Optimum Nutrition
5 Jerdan Place, London SW6 1BE

Cover Design : QA

ISBN 1 87097 602 9

Printed and bound in Great Britain by
Brier Press, High Wycombe, Bucks

CONTENTS

ABOUT THE AUTHOR

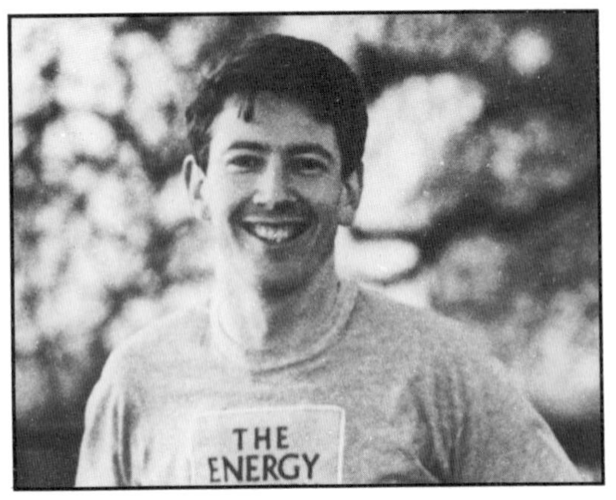

Patrick Holford started his career in the field of psychology where he researched ways of maximising mental health. His research led him into the field of nutrition which has been his speciality since 1979. In 1984 he founded the Institute for Optimum Nutrition, an independent centre for the research and practice of nutrition, of which he is a co-director. His time is divided between teaching and training nutritionists, seeing clients, writing and researching.

He is author of many popular nutrition books including The Whole Health Manual, Elemental Health, Vitamin Vitality, The Metabolic Diet, The Better Pregnancy Diet, The Energy Equation and The Family Nutrition Workbook, writes for a number of national magazines and newspapers and frequently appears on radio and television.

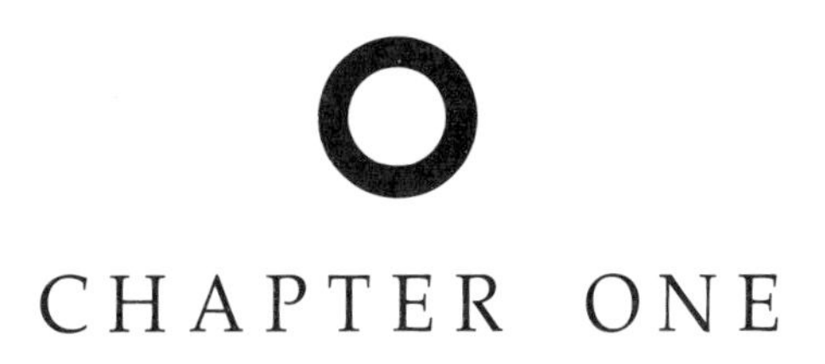

CHAPTER ONE

HEART DISEASE – THE MODERN EPIDEMIC

ONE in two men and women die from heart disease. Currently 125,000 people die prematurely from a stroke or heart attack. One man in four will have a heart attack before retirement age and one quarter of deaths occur in people under the age of 65. For women, heart disease and strokes are second only to cancer as the leading cause of death between the ages of 35 and 54. While heart disease usually strikes after the age of 45 even by the age of 10, fatty deposits which herald the beginning of arterial disease are already present in most people's arteries. So widespread is this modern epidemic of heart disease that we almost take it for granted. We fail to protect ourselves from a disease, whose cause, for the large part is known, and whose cure is already proven, a disease more life threatening than AIDS. According to the US Surgeon General, of the 2.2 million Americans who die each year, no less than 1.6 million die from diet related diseases, predominantly of the heart and arteries. This book is, quite simply, essential for anyone interested in living. I predict that following the advice in this book is likely to add at least ten years to your healthy lifespan.

There is nothing natural about dying from heart disease. Many cultures in the world do not experience the high incidence of strokes or heart attacks. For example, by middle age British people have nine times as much heart disease as the Japanese. Autopsies performed on Egyptian mummies dying in 3000 B.C. show signs of deposits in the arteries but no actual blockages that result in a stroke or heart attack. Despite the obvious signs of a heart attack (severe chest pain, cold sweats, nausea, fall in blood pressure and weak pulse) in the 1930's a heart attack was so rare that it took a specialist to make the diagnosis. According to American health records the incidence per 100,000 people of heart attack was none in 1890 and had risen to 340 by 1970. Although deaths did occur from other forms of heart disease including calcified valves, rheumatic heart and other congenital defects, the incidence of actual blockages in the arteries causing a stroke or heart attack was minimal. Even more concerning is the fact that heart disease is occurring earlier and earlier. Autopsies performed in Vietnam showed that one in two soldiers killed in action, with an average age of 22, already had atherosclerosis. Nowadays most teenagers can be expected to show signs of atherosclerosis, heralding the beginning of heart disease. Obviously something about our lifestyle, diet or environment has changed radically in the last sixty years to bring on this modern epidemic.

WHAT IS HEART DISEASE?

The cardiovascular system consists of blood vessels that carry oxygen, fuel (glucose), building materials (amino acids), vitamins and minerals to every single cell in your body. The blood is oxygenated when tiny blood vessels, called capillaries, absorb oxygen from the lungs, and in turn discharge carbon dioxide, which we then exhale. These blood vessels feed into the heart which pumps the oxygenated blood to all cells. At the cells the blood vessels once more become a network of extremely thin capillaries which give off oxygen plus other

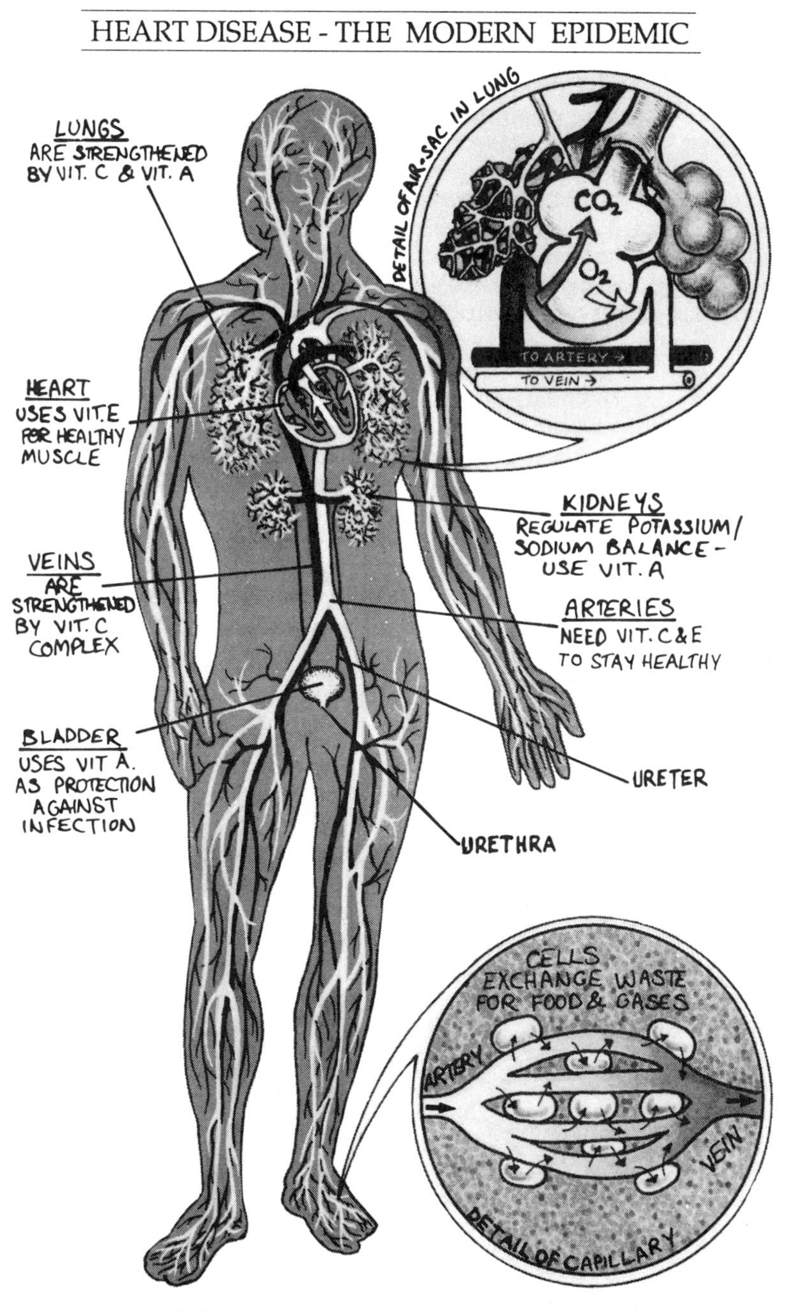

DIAGRAM 1 - The Cardiovascular System

nutrients and can receive waste products from these cells. Oxygen plus glucose is needed to make energy within every cell, from brain cells to muscle cells. The waste products are carbon dioxide and water, which are returned into the capillaries. Blood vessels supplying cells with nutrients and oxygen are called arteries, while blood vessels carrying away waste products and carbon dioxide are called veins. Arterial blood is redder because oxygen is carried on a complex called haemoglobin, which contains iron. The pressure in the arteries is also greater than in the veins. As well as returning to the heart all blood passes through the kidneys. Here, waste products are removed, and formed into urine which stores in the bladder.

Heart disease is wrongly named. The main life-threatening diseases are diseases of the arteries. Over a number of years changes can occur within the artery walls that lead to deposition of unwanted substances, including cholesterol, other fats and calcium. This is called arterial plaque, or an *atheroma* from the greek word for porridge, because of the porridge like consistency of these deposits. The presence of arterial deposits is called *atherosclerosis.* Atherosclerosis occurs in very particular parts of the body shown in the diagram opposite. The presence of atherosclerosis, coupled with thicker blood containing blood clots, can lead to a blockage in the artery, stopping blood flow. If this occurs in the arteries feeding the heart the part of the heart fed by these blood vessels will die from a lack of oxygen. This is called a *myocardial infarction* or heart attack. Before this occurs many people are diagnosed as having *angina,* a condition in which there is a limited supply of oxygen to the heart due to partial blockage of coronary arteries, causing chest pain, most classically on exertion or when under stress.

If a blockage occurs in the brain, part of the brain dies. This is called a stroke. The arteries in the brain are especially fragile and sometimes a stroke occurs not as a result of a blockage but because an artery ruptures. This is called a *cerebral haemorrhage.* If a blockage occurs in the legs this can result in leg pain, which is a form of *thrombosis* (a thrombus is a blood clot). When peripheral arteries get blocked this can result in poor peripheral circulation.

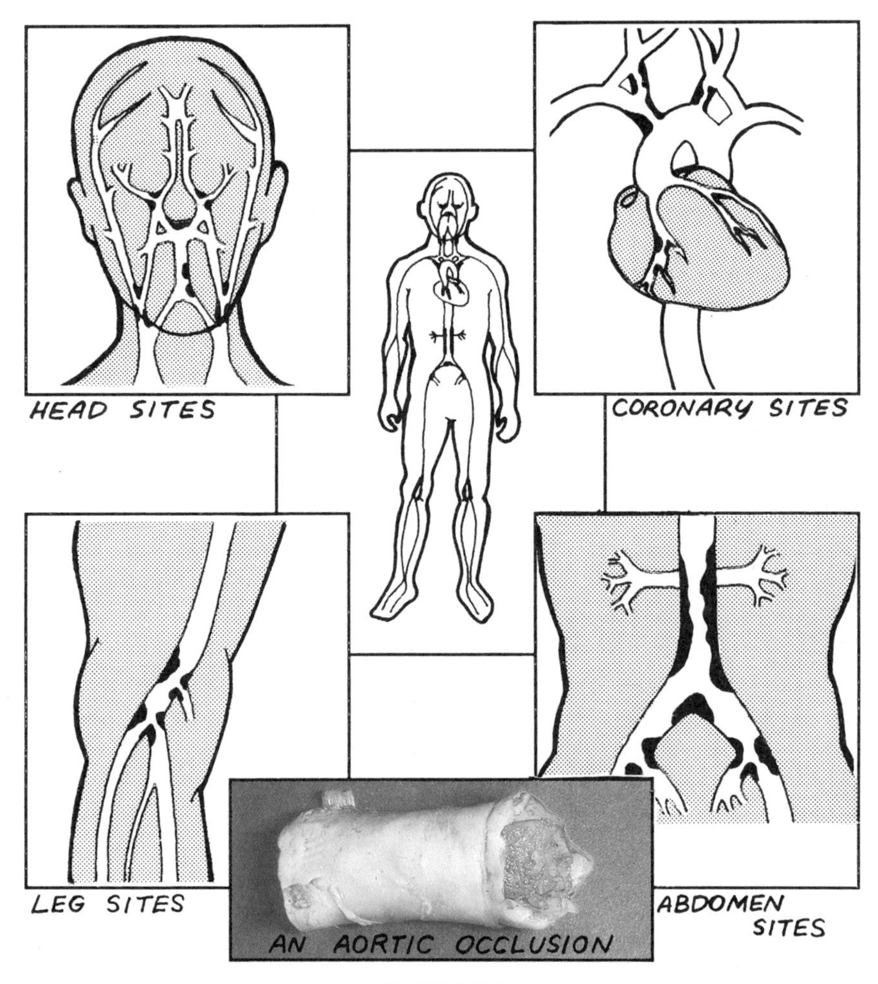

- DIAGRAM 2 -

COMMON SITES OF ATHEROSCLEROTIC LESIONS

UNDERSTANDING BLOOD PRESSURE

So two main factors are responsible for so-called heart disease. Atherosclerosis, the formation of deposits, and the presence of blood clots, thick blood. However there is a third problem that can and usually does occur along with atherosclerosis. That is *arteriosclerosis,* the hardening of the arteries. Arteries are elastic, and whether or not atherosclerosis is present, tend to harden with age. One reason this can occur is due to a lack of vitamin C which is needed to make collagen, the intercellular glue that keeps skin and arteries supple. Arteriosclerosis, atherosclerosis and thick blood can all raise blood pressure.

Imagine a hosepipe attached to a tap that turns on and off. When the tap is on the pressure is greatest, and when the tap is off the pressure is lowest. That's what blood pressure is all about. A blood pressure of 120/80 means that the maximum pressure when the heart has just beaten is 120 units, and the minimum pressure when the heart is in a lull, is 80 units. Imagine if the hosepipe was metal rather than rubber. This would raise the pressure wouldn't it? If the hosepipe was furred up, or if the fluid was thicker these too would raise the pressure. So a raised blood pressure is a reliable indication that all is not right. Life insurance companies rely heavily on blood pressure to predict expected lifespan.

A blood pressure of 120/80 or less is ideal. A top figure (the *systolic* pressure) of more than 140, or a bottom figure (the *diastolic* pressure) of more than 90 indicates a potential problem. A blood pressure of 150/100 indicates a serious risk of heart disease. For example, a 55 year old man with a blood pressure of 120/80, will, on average, live to the age of 78. A 55 year old man with a blood pressure of 150/100 is predicted to live to 72. High blood pressure, called *hypertension* , is a silent killer. Only one in ten people with raised blood pressure are aware of it. After the age of 25 most people's blood pressure increases quite rapidly. So a yearly blood pressure check is always recommended. If you're healthy there's no reason why your blood pressure should increase with age. Many 'primitive' cultures show no increase in blood pressure with age.

WHAT CAUSES HEART DISEASE?

Back in 1913 a Russian scientist Dr. Anitschkov, thought he had found the answer to heart disease. He found that feeding cholesterol to rabbits induced heart disease. He failed to realise that rabbits, being vegetarians, have no means for dealing with this animal fat.

Since the fatty deposits in the arteries of people with heart disease have also been found to be high in cholesterol, it was soon thought that these deposits were the result of an excess of cholesterol in the blood, possibly caused by an excess of cholesterol in the diet.

Such a simple theory had its attractions and many doctors still advocate a low cholesterol diet as the answer to heart disease - despite a consistent lack of results. If the cholesterol theory was correct, we would expect that: people with high dietary cholesterol would have a high incidence of heart disease; raising dietary cholesterol would raise blood cholesterol; and blood cholesterol levels would be good predictors of heart disease.

THE CHOLESTEROL MYTH

Dr Alfin-Slater from the University of California decided to test the cholesterol theory. "We, like everyone else, had been convinced that when you eat cholesterol you get cholesterol. When we stopped to think, none of the studies in the past had tested what happens to cholesterol levels when eggs, high in cholesterol, were added to a normal diet."

They selected 50 healthy people with normal blood cholesterol levels. Half of them were given two eggs per day (in addition to the other cholesterol rich foods they were already eating as part of their normal diet) for eight weeks. The other half were given one extra egg per day for four weeks, then two extra eggs per day for the next four weeks. The results showed no change in blood cholesterol. Later, Dr Alfin Slater commented "Our findings surprised us as much as ever..."

Three other studies (Professor Ismail, 1976; Dr.Hirshowitz, 1976; Dr. Herbert, 1977) have also found no rise in blood cholesterol levels. In fact, as long ago as 1974, a British advisory panel set up by the government to look at 'medical aspects of food policy on diet related to cardio-vascular disease' issued this statement: "Most of the dietary cholesterol in Western communities is derived from eggs, but we have found no evidence which relates the number of eggs consumed to heart disease."

During the height of cholesterol phobia, Dr. Jolliffe, renowned for his weight reducing diets, started an 'anti-coronary club' and placed 814 men, aged 40 to 59, all free from heart disease, on a low cholesterol, high polyunsaturated fat diet. For a control group he had 463 men of similar age and health status, who continued with a normal, and thus relatively high cholesterol diet. Five years later, eight men on the low cholesterol diet had died from heart attacks, compared to none in the control group! Ironically, Dr. Jolliffe himself died from vascular complications of diabetes at the age of 59, so he never lived to see the results.

IS FAT TO BLAME?

As scientists became disillusioned with the cholesterol diets their attention turned to saturated fat. After all, eating too much fat leads to obesity and the incidence of heart disease in obese people is twice as high. Too much saturated fat raises levels of triglycerides (the official word for fat in the blood) and also blood cholesterol, both of which are good indicators of a high risk. Also, the fatty streaks and deposits that occur in arteries are high in triglycerides. In Western society, although not in some primitive societies, a high saturated fat intake is associated with increased risk of heart disease.

However, simply substituting saturated fats, generally found in meat, for poly-unsaturated fats, found in vegetables, nuts and seeds, is also not the answer. In some studies raising poly-unsaturated fat intake actually raised blood cholesterol levels! The answer, at least as far as fat is concerned, is to cut down the overall intake of saturated fat by eating less meat and fatty dairy products.

There is little doubt that too much fat is a major factor in heart disease, but it is not the only one. After all, Eskimos, who eat a high saturated fat and cholesterol diet, have the lowest incidence of heart disease. So if heart disease isn't predominantly caused by eating too much cholesterol or saturated fat what is it caused by?

HEART DISEASE - THE NEW THEORY

The 'furring up' of arteries is far more complex than just a simple deposition of fats. While the whole process still isn't completely understood it appears that damage occurs in three phases.

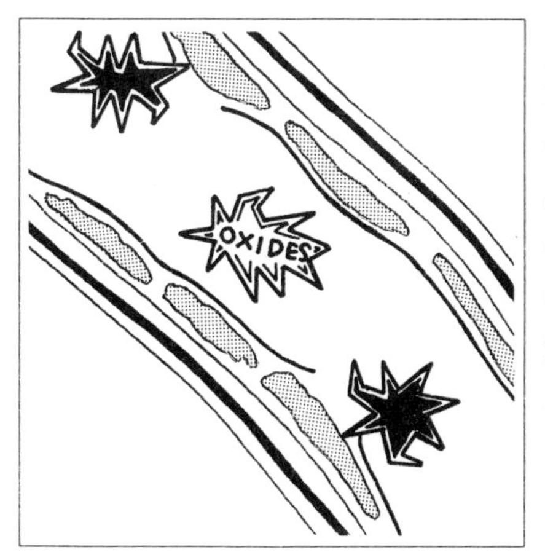

Phase 1 - The Artery Wall Gets Damaged - This can be caused by dangerous by-products of oxygen called oxides. These are created when fat is fried, and are present in cigarette smoke and anything burnt like barbecued or smoked food, as well as in car fumes and the 'used' air we expel.

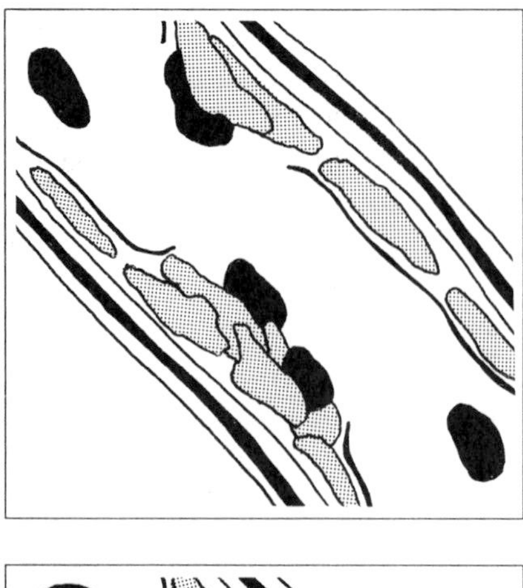

Phase 2 - The Cells Proliferate - Perhaps as an attempt to effect repair, cells in the artery wall begin to proliferate much like cancer cells. They also behave incorrectly accumulating excess cholesterol from the blood stream. The growing deposit also attracts calcium and other fats present in the blood. If there is an excess of cholesterol or fat in the blood the whole process speeds up.

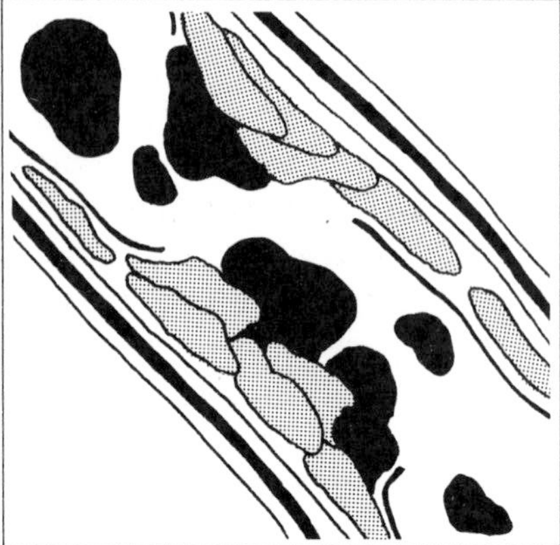

Phase 3 - The Blockage Develops - By now the artery is already substantially restricted in circumference. If the blood itself is thick and contains blood clots, or if a deposit breaks off from another part of the artery wall, this can result in a total blockage of the artery.

The inside of our arteries represent a very large surface area along which rushes blood at high pressure. Just like our skin we are prone to the odd cut or bruise. This damage is most likely to be caused by free radicals, which are incomplete oxygen molecules that have an uneven electrical charge. Just like a magnet attracts metal objects these free radicals attack cell walls and the nucleus of cells, in an attempt to restore its electrical balance. This can lead to cell death, an inability to control what comes into the cell, and replication of the cell itself. There is evidence that all of these things happen in the cells in the artery walls. As some of these cells die, greater amounts of cholesterol and fat enters through the cell wall. The cells within the artery wall become full of fat and cholesterol and other debris used by the body to attempt to repair the wound. Within atheromas are also found identical cells. This led to the discovery by Dr Benditt and his team in 1973 that cells within atheromas were actually multiplying much like cancer cells. These new cells not only store cholesterol and other material, but also produce it. As the atheroma becomes larger even more cholesterol and calcium are electrically attracted to it, a process which is entirely independent of the concentration of calcium or cholesterol in the blood. The addition of calcium hardens the atheroma.

Even though the initial process that causes cellular damage may have little to do with excess fat or cholesterol it is the on-going accumulation of cholesterol and fat that leads to the development of larger and larger atheromas. It is worth, therefore, taking a closer look at how the body controls blood cholesterol levels. Cholesterol is essential to the human body. It is needed for nerve transmission, it is converted into various hormones including sex hormones and is incorporated into various cell membranes particularly in the brain. It is also a constituent of bile, a substance produced by the liver which helps to break down and digest fats. Blood vessels themselves produce cholesterol to provide lubrication. Cholesterol can be made from protein, fats or carbohydrates. If you were to completely avoid eating cholesterol your body would still produce enough for all these functions.

In order to be carried around the body cholesterol becomes bound to a type of protein called a lipoprotein. Usually around 70 per cent of cholesterol in the blood is carried in the form of low density lipoproteins (LDLs). The rest is carried in the form of high density lipoproteins (HDLs). While LDLs help to transport cholesterol into cells, HDLs help remove cholesterol from the blood and from artery walls and return it to the liver where it can be formed into bile, a small amount of which is then excreted via the digestive system. Eskimos, who have a very high saturated fat and cholesterol diet also have high HDL levels and virtually no cardiovascular disease. The most likely reason for this is their high consumption of a particular fatty acid called EPA (discussed later) which encourages HDLs. However other nutrients also help to control what the body does with cholesterol.

With this new model of the causes of heart disease it is easy to see how there are many risk factors for cardiovascular disease, from smoking which encourages initial artery wall damage by creating free radicals, to stress or lack of exercise, which raise blood pressure, and excess consumption of saturated fat, which encourages the development of atherosclerotic deposits. There are also many ways, both through diet and lifestyle to make sure that these unwelcome changes do not happen to your arteries by, for example, decreasing your intake of substances that introduce free radicals to the body; increasing your intake of anti-oxidant nutrients like vitamin E that disarm free radicals; increasing your intake of nutrients, like EPA, that encourage proper control of circulating cholesterol; all quite apart from the obvious advice of cutting down fat intake and keeping fit.

The next chapter explains what all the risk factors are, shows you how to work out your risk and the areas in your diet and lifestyle that will make the most difference to the health of your heart and arteries.

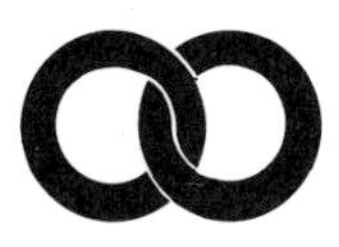

CHAPTER TWO

HOW HEALTHY IS YOUR HEART?

DESPITE differing opinions about the cause and treatment of heart disease one thing is certain. There are many contributive causes, two of which are a lack of exercise and faulty nutrition. Both have been shown to help, but neither provide all the answers. Jim Fix, the famous author of the Complete Book of Running, died at the age of 52 from a heart attack while jogging. The autopsy found that two of his coronary arteries were almost totally clogged, which is not surprising to those who know of his disregard for dietary advice. On the other hand, the heart surgeon, Dr Albert Starr, an advocator and follower of the low cholesterol diet, needed open-heart surgery at only 47 years of age, the very same operation he had performed over 3,000 times! In an experiment designed to determine which is more important - diet or exercise - Bill Solomon, from the University of Arizona, got some obliging pigs to run around a track, but fed them the average vitamin-deficient diet. Another group ate the pig-equivalent of health food but had no exercise; and a third group had both exercise *and* good nutrition. The third group of pigs fared best, proving that exercise and good nutrition together are vital for a healthy heart.

WHAT ARE THE RISK FACTORS?

These are shown in the table below. You don't have to have all of them to be at risk. Smoking a little, drinking a little, exercising too little, eating a little too much fat and not enough protective vitamins and minerals can be as bad as smoking a lot, or drinking a lot, provided other areas of your health are well covered. Later on in this chapter you'll be able to assess your overall risk and see clearly which changes to your diet and lifestyle will make the most difference to the health of your cardiovascular system. Before assessing your risk it is best to understand why these factors are important.

HEART DISEASE - What Are the Risk Factors?

Lack of exercise
Excessive stress
Smoking
Excessive alcohol consumption
High blood lipids (cholesterol, triglycerides)
High blood pressure
Too much salt
Too much sugar and fat
Too little fibre
Low intake of vitamins, especially C and E
Low intake of minerals, especially Magnesium and Selenium
Family history of heart disease or diabetes

Exercise Prevents Heart Disease

Human beings are designed to exercise. Just being sedentary *doubles* your risk for heart disease. Even moderate exercise two or three times a week has been shown to raise high density lipoproteins, lower cholesterol and blood pressure. The more you exercise the stronger is the effect. But not all forms of exercise help. The most health promoting are 'aerobic' exercises such as jogging, swimming, cycling and brisk walking. If you consider yourself unfit you'll need to start gently, perhaps exercising twice a week, for half an hour. It's good to get some advice from a professional, so you don't start off with too ambitious an aim, only to give up after a couple of weeks.

Stress Promotes It

Stress promotes high blood pressure. This is a natural consequence of our evolution. Our primate ancestors, when under stress, needed to 'fight or take flight'. One component of the many changes that occur is a raised blood pressure necessary for the extreme muscular activity needed to fight or run. Another is thickening blood, which would have helped heal wounds. Nowadays our stresses are different and impossible to avoid completely. Prolonged stress increases your risk for heart disease. Although it isn't that easy to do, reducing stress and learning how to relax make a difference. If you can't avoid stress then it's doubly important to make sure your nutrition is up to scratch.

Smoking Increases Your Risk by 70%!

Smoking a packet of cigarettes a day gives you twice the risk of a heart attack and five times the risk of a stroke. Smoking 40 cigarettes a day means you are five times more likely to die of heart disease. In Britain thirty thousand people die of heart disease directly as a result of smoking. The two major toxins in cigarettes are carbon monoxide and nicotine. Both increase blood clotting, promote artery damage and the formation of clots. Cigarettes also cause a restriction of blood vessels, therefore raising blood pressure. Nine out of ten heavy smokers have moderate to advanced atherosclerosis compared to three in ten non-smokers.

Alcohol - A little is Good, A lot is Bad

You may be surprised to hear that small amounts of alcohol may actually be good for you. Studies have shown that a small daily intake of alcohol actually raises levels of high density lipoproteins, which help to return cholesterol to the liver from where it can be excreted. This effect soon vanishes once more than two ounces of alcohol are consumed. So a maximum of two glasses of wine, two beers or two measures of whisky, for example, *may* be beneficial. However, even small amounts of alcohol seem to raise blood pressure. A group of researchers wondered why people going into hospital tended to have a drop in blood pressure. Thinking that the reduction in alcohol consumption might have something to do with it, they equipped a new group of patients with a complementary daily can of beer. Sure enough, these patients didn't show the usual decline in blood pressure. Alcohol, being a neuro-toxin, and a substance which robs the body of both vitamins and minerals, can hardly be recommended for improving your health. However, a drink a day, at least from the point of heart disease, probably has little effect.

What's Your Cholesterol Level?

The best predictor of heart disease is the level of cholesterol and triglycerides in the blood. In order to be carried in the blood, cholesterol becomes bound to a type of protein called a *lipoprotein*. Usually around 70 per cent of the cholesterol in the blood is carried in the form of low density lipoproteins (LDLs). The rest is carried in the form of high density lipoproteins (HDLs). As overall blood cholesterol levels rise, so does the amount of LDLs, both of which indicate an increased risk for cardiovascular disease. HDLs, on the other hand, seem to help remove cholesterol from the blood and from artery walls and return it to the liver, where it can be formed into bile and excreted via the digestive system. So a raised HDL level is broadly speaking consistent with a reduced risk. The best predictor is the ratio between HDL levels and cholesterol. These are shown in the chart below.

YOUR IDEAL BLOOD FAT LEVELS

RISK	LOW RISK	MEDIUM	HIGH
CHOLESTEROL	<5.18	6.2	>6.7
TRIGLYCERIDES	<1.0	1.5	>1.95
HDLs	>0.91	0.7	<0.5
CHOLESTEROL/HDLS	3:1	5:1	8:1

(All measurements in MMOL/Litre)

A high level of triglycerides (which just means fat) in the blood also indicates an increased risk. When triglycerides are raised but cholesterol is not this can indicate an excessive intake of sugar and other refined carbohydrates.

Your Pulse and Blood Pressure

Your pulse and blood pressure are the easiest way to get some insight into the health of your cardiovascular system. Your pulse reflects the strength of your heart. If your heart only has to beat 60 times each minute to get the blood circluating around your body it is obviously healthier than if your heart has to beat 80 times a minute. The more you exercise the stronger your heart, which is, after all, just a muscle, becomes. Cyclists have very large hearts while sedentary people have small hearts. The ideal pulse rate is below 65 beats a minute. Some athletes have pulse rates as low as 45, however, for most people to get your pulse down to sixty is the most one can hope for.

Your blood pressure reflects the health of your arteries more than the health of your heart. The higher your blood pressure the more likely you are to have atherosclerosis and the greater is your risk for cardiovascular disease. Generally speaking a systolic pressure above 140, or a diastolic pressure above 90 indicates a significant risk for heart disease. The table below shows you what your ideal blood pressure and pulse should be.

YOUR IDEAL PULSE AND BLOOD PRESSURE

	LOW RISK	MEDIUM	HIGH RISK
PULSE	60-69	70-79	80 +
BLOOD PRESSURE	90/60 to 125/85	126/86 to 135/89	136/90 or higher

Are you Pickling Yourself with Salt?

Salt is a preservative. It first came into use to preserve meat by slowing down the enzyme reactions that cause meat to decay. Although we need to take in some salt every day it is present in all foods, including fruit and vegetables. There is simply no need to add it to your diet. The excessive consumption of salt is known to raise blood pressure, especially in susceptible individuals. Unfortunately, there is no easy way to determine whether or not you are particularly susceptible to the effects of salt so the best advice is to avoid added salt. The average person consumes over 10 grams a day which is more than twenty times our actual requirement. For most people, avoiding salt makes a measurable difference to blood pressure.

The three S's - Sugar, Saturated Fat and Stimulants

Sugar consumption is associated with both raised blood pressure and an increased incidence of cardiovascular disease. Some researchers even consider it to be more important than the consumption of fat. Sugar increased blood stickiness which can lead to the formation of clots. If the extra sugar is not required it is converted into fat. A high sugar diet raises your blood pressure, decreases your resistance to stress, another risk factor, and is associated with diabetes. Since most diabetics develop cardiovascular disease the association between sugar and refined carbohydrates and heart disease is very strong. Conversely, a diet high in fibre and complex carbohydrates such as lentils, beans and wholegrains decreases your risk.

Sugar acts as a stimulant. It can induce bursts of hyperactivity followed by a slump in energy. So can other stimulants like chocolate, cola drinks, coffee and tea, which stimulate the body to release sugar stores. Coffee and tea deplete the body of minerals, including potassium and magnesium, both by decreasing their absorption and by promoting their excretion via the kidneys. Your overall intake of stimulants increases your risk for cardiovascular disease.

Fat makes up 42 per cent of the calories of the average diet. Nearly half the fat we consume is saturated. Saturated fat is not a necessary component in our diets even though it is impossible and unnecessary to completely avoid it. It can be turned into glucose for energy or stored as fat which at least keeps us insulated and gives us padding. It is consistent with health to cut down overall intake to 30 per cent of total calories, with saturated fat making up no more than a third of total fat intake. The old advice of switching from saturated fats to poly-unsaturated fats, by, for example, eating margarine rather than butter, is not recommended. A high poly-unsaturated fat intake is also not good. Poly-unsaturated fats, primarily when cooked or processed, lead to the formation of free radicals. So the message is to cut down on overall fat intake by having skimmed milk, becoming semi-vegetarian and eating fish and chicken instead of meat, having less cheese and avoiding junk and heavily processed food which are usually full of sugar and saturated fat. Foods rich in poly-unsaturated fats are beneficial to the body and are best eaten raw. So keep your cold-pressed vegetable oils for salad dressings and mayonnaise, eat nuts and seeds and avoid frying as much as you can.

Vitamins and Minerals

The role of certain micronutrients, vitamins, minerals and essential fatty acids, in preventing cardiovascular disease is greatly underestimated. It is hard to predict to what extent the decline in our intake of vitamins and minerals has been responsible, for the increase in cardiovascular disease. A good supply of anti-oxidant nutrients, which protect the body from harmful free radicals that damage cells in the artery wall, is essential. Vitamin A, both retinol, the animal form, and beta-carotene, the vegetable form, vitamin C and E all act as anti-oxidants. Other anti-oxidant enzymes depend upon selenium, zinc, manganese and iron. The most important of these are vitamins A, C and E and selenium. Vitamin B6 deficiency is also associated with cardiovascular disease. Although the exact mechanism is not fully understood Vitamin B6 is needed to make lecithin which is essential for normal cholesterol metabolism. Blood pressure can be lowered by ensuring a good intake of calcium, magnesium and potassium. Of these magnesium is the most important nutrient. The role all these nutrients play in preventing cardiovascular disease is explained fully, together with recommended intakes, in the next chapter.

What Have You Inherited?

If heart disease or diabetes runs in your family this immediately increases your risk. One reason for this is passed on negative dietary and lifestyle habits, however it appears that there is a genetic component to our inherited high risk. Although there's nothing you can do to change the past what you can do is to protect your future by following the advice in this book.

THE HEALTHY HEART CHECK

The following questionnaire is designed to let you assess how you rate on each of the major risk factors. The central diagram represents the diameter of an artery. For each point you score, shade in one of the blocks starting at the outside, to see at a glance your risk for heart disease. The greater your risk the smaller the diameter of the artery, giving less room for the blood to flow and a higher risk of blockages.

Exercise Check

Colour in one section in the exercise sector for each NO answer

a) Do you take exercise that noticeably raises your heartbeat for more than 20 minutes, three or more times a week?

b) Does your job involve lots of walking, lifting or vigorous activity?

c) Do you regularly play an active sport?

d) Do you have any physically tiring hobbies?

e) Do you consider yourself physically fit?

Stress Check

Colour in one section in the stress sector for each YES answer

a) Do you feel guilty when relaxing?

b) Do you have a persistent need for recognition or achievement or are you especially competitive?

c) Do you work harder than most or do you often do two or more tasks at a time?

d) Do you easily become angry or impatient if things hold you up?

e) Do you find it difficult to openly admit defeat?

Smoking Check

Colour in one section in the smoking sector for each YES answer

a) Do you smoke 1 - 10 cigarettes a day?

b) Do you smoke more than 10 cigarettes a day?

c) More than 15?

d) More than 20?

e) Do you smoke a pipe or cigars?

Stimulant Check

Colour in one section in the stimulant sector for each YES answer

a) Do you drink more than four cups of coffee a day?
b) Do you drink more than six cups of tea a day?
c) Do you have more than three alcoholic drinks a day?
d) Do you often eat chocolate more than three times a week?
e) Do you add sugar to food or drink every day?

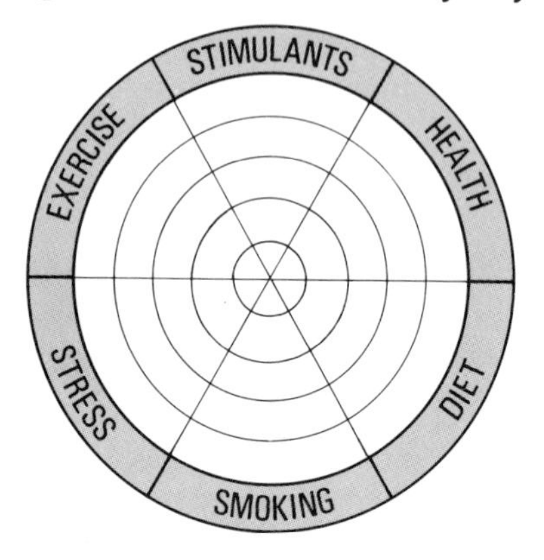

Health Check

Colour in one section in the health sector for each YES answer

a) Is your pulse over 90 beats per minute?
b) Have you ever had high blood pressure?
c) Have either of your parents ever had high blood pressure or diabetes?
d) Is there a broader family history of heart disease or diabetes?

Diet Check

a) Do you use salt when cooking and add it to your food?
b) Do you eat fried food more than twice a week?
c) Do you eat white bread or rice and processed foods more often than whole grains, lentils or beans?
d) Do you eat red meat more than twice a week?
e) Does less than a third of your diet consist of raw fruit and vegetables?

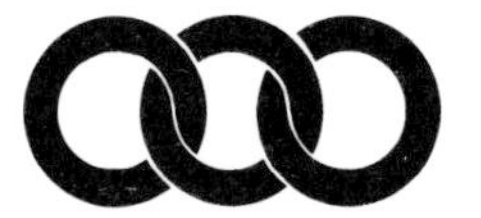

CHAPTER THREE

SUPERNUTRITION FOR A HEALTHY HEART

NOW that you know what the risk factors are and what heart disease is all about what can you do to prevent it? Obviously you can minimise your risk by avoiding smoking, reducing your fat intake, exercising more and decreasing other risk factors. There are also many ways, through optimum nutrition that you can further protect yourself.

The first step is to protect your arteries from the initial damage that leads to the development of atherosclerosis and ensure that your arteries can heal themselves when damage does occur.

PROTECTING YOUR ARTERIES

The primary cause of arterial damage is from free radicals. These are incomplete molecules containing oxygen which have an uneven electrical charge. All stable atoms and collections of atoms, called molecules, have an even electrical charge. Free radicals don't so they try to complete themselves by robbing neighbouring cells. This can set up a chain reaction of damage until the free radical is disarmed by an anti-oxidant, for example, vitamin C. Free radicals attack double bonds which are found in greatest supply in fats and in the DNA molecule. The walls of cells, including those in the arteries, incorporate fats to give them flexibility, and therefore contain double bonds. The nucleus of the cell contains DNA which provides the code for proper cell behaviour. So free radicals tend to destroy cell walls and damage the nucleus of cells. This affects the supply of nutrients to the cell and may lead to the excessive accumulation of unwanted substances, such as cholesterol. If the cell nucleus is damaged the cell won't carry out its functions properly and may start to multiply, which is how cancer starts.

We obtain free radicals from many sources. Any combustion process creates free radicals, so car exhaust and factory fumes all give us a generous supply of free radicals. The sun's rays also generate free radicals which is why people living in hot countries are more prone to skin cancer. Heated fats, especially unsaturated fats, generate free radicals. The more unsaturated the fat or oil the more free radicals are created. So if you do fry foods it is best to use butter or olive oil, which is mono-unsaturated, not cold-pressed sunflower oil, which is poly-unsaturated. However it is best to avoid frying as much as possible in favour of grilling or baking. Anything burnt creates free radicals. That includes toast, barbecues, smoked food and cigarettes.

Free radicals are not completely avoidable. We actually produce them as a result of making energy from 'burning' glucose with oxygen. They can be thought of as our 'nuclear waste' - rather hard to dispose of. But they can be disposed of by the body's anti-oxidant systems. Vitamin A, both in the animal form of retinol, and in the vegetable form of beta-carotene, acts as an anti-oxidant. Ideally one should obtain both forms. Beta-carotene is rich in all red-yellow vegetables and fruits including carrots, tomatoes, beetroot, watermelon and apricots. Carrots are the richest source and a carrot a day is an excellent way to up

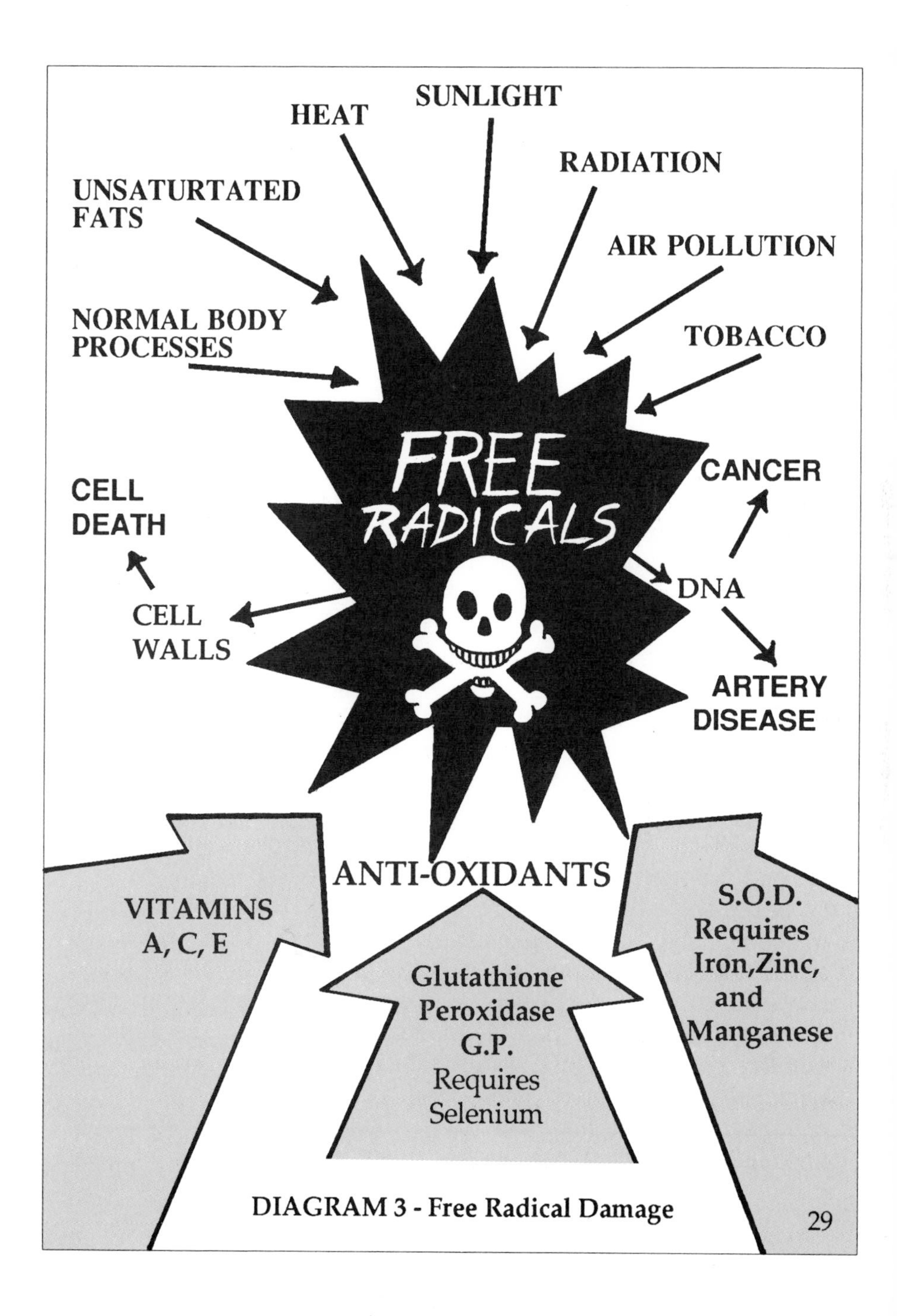

DIAGRAM 3 - Free Radical Damage

your intake of this valuable nutrient. Probably the ideal intake of vitamin A is in the region of 40,000iu's per day. This is roughly equivalent to what our ancestors would have eaten. Most of this comes from beta-carotene which is non-toxic. One can safely assume that a diet high in fruit and vegetables can provide 20,000iu's, so a general recommendation would be to supplement 7,500iu's of retinol and 12,500iu's of beta-carotene, making a total of 20,000iu's per day from supplements, plus 20,000iu's from diet.

Vitamin C is an all-rounder as far as artery protection is concerned. Low levels of vitamin C are found in individuals prone to heart attack and the lower the level the less chance they have of surviving a heart attack. It is thought that whatever available vitamin C there is collects in the heart to help repair the damage leaving blood levels low. Vitamin C is an anti-oxidant and also potentiates the anti-oxidant effect of vitamin E. It is also required to keep artery walls healthy. A lack of vitamin C makes artery walls abnormally permeable. This is because vitamin C is required to make collagen, which acts like intercellular glue.

Most significant of all is evidence that vitamin C helps to reverse plaque formation and remove cholesterol from the arteries. People who are deficient in this vitamin are more prone to plaque formation and are less able to convert unwanted cholesterol into bile. Vitamin C appears to lower, or at least normalise cholesterol levels and raise HDLs which help to escort cholesterol away. So does vitamin B3 (in the niacin or nicotinic acid form). However, in people with advanced atherosclerosis vitamin C can temporarily increase blood cholesterol levels as cholesterol is removed from plaques later to be escorted from the bloodstream. It is best therefore to monitor cholesterol/HDL ratios which are a better predictor of what is happening to cholesterol. If vitamin C didn't do enough already it has also been shown to reduce blood clot formation. Everyone can benefit from supplementing at least

1,000mg (1 gram) of vitamin C a day.

Vitamin E is the most important vitamin for promoting cardiovascular health. It's list of beneficial actions is a long one. Firstly, vitamin E acts as an anti-oxidant. It also helps cells to use oxygen. This is particularly important for people with angina, where the supply of oxygen to the heart is impaired, or for those who have recently had a heart attack or stroke. One study showed that angina patients supplementing 400iu's of vitamin E a day were able to reduce their nitroglycerine medication.

PREVENTING BLOOD CLOTS WITH VITAMIN E

However the most important asset of vitamin E is its ability to dissolve existing blood clots and keep the blood thin. This effect has been known for the last forty years yet vitamin E is still not recommended in place of anti-coagulant drugs. Many anti-coagulant drugs, including heparin and aspirin, have the disadvantage of promoting bleeding. Vitamin E does not.

If you are taking anti-coagulant drugs you should not greatly increase your intake of vitamin E above 200iu's without first checking with your doctor as the combination of certain drugs and vitamin E can lead to an unnaturally prolonged clotting time. There is, however, no danger in supplementing vitamin E on its own. If you have a history of heart disease or high blood pressure it is best to increase your vitamin E intake gradually, by 100ius per month, up to a maximum of 1,000ius.

The blood forms clots because plate-shaped substances called platelets form a clump. Platelets stick to collagen produced by the smooth muscle cells that multiply in atheromas. Your blood clotting tendency can be measured by determining your *platelet adhesion index* . A normal platelet adhesion index would be 20 to 35. People who have just had a heart attack may have an index of 90 or more, while those prone to heart attacks often have an index over 50. Many drugs do not effect platelet clotting, but rather blood clotting at a later stage. Vitamin E (and EPA) effectively reduce platelet adhesion which is the very basis of blood clotting and the formation of blood clots which represent a real danger if arteries are already partially blocked.

There is little doubt that vitamin E supplementation reduces the risk of heart attack and increases the health of your heart and arteries. Everyone can benefit from supplementing 200iu's of vitamin E a day, although in people with cardiovascular disease levels up to 1,000iu's may be more beneficial. However, it is best to start with a smaller amount and increase gradually.

EPA - THE ESKIMO SECRET

Eskimos have always been an enigma as far as heart disease is concerned. First we had the cholesterol theory, but Eskimos eat tons of cholesterol and rarely suffer from heart disease. Then we had the theory that too much fat causes heart disease. Once again Eskimos put a spanner in the works with their incredibly high fat intake from fatty fish. Dr. Hugh Sinclair, one of Britain's most respected medical researchers, determined in 1954 to solve the riddle of the Eskimos.

His researcher confirmed experience from Japan that a diet high in cold water fish, like salmon, herring, mackerel, haddock or sardines protected against heart disease. But what was it in the fish that protected against heart disease and how did it work? The answer was a special kind of fat, *eicosapentaenoic acid* , or EPA for short.

Five properly controlled medical studies, from Canada, America, England, Denmark and Japan, have all confirmed that EPA does a lot to combat heart disease. It lowers blood pressure, blood fats and cholesterol and raises HDLs, the cholesterol scavenger. It also thins the blood by reducing the platelet adhesion index. No drug yet developed has so complete an effect as this natural nutrient in reducing these markers of heart disease. Dr William Connors, professor of medicine at the

University of Oregon, found that a ten day diet of salmon, containing large amounts of EPA, lowered cholesterol levels by 17 per cent in healthy people and 20 per cent in those with raised cholesterol. Triglyceride levels fell by up to 67 per cent! "The greatest effect seems to be with patients with elevation of both cholesterol and triglyceride levels." says Dr Connor, "The higher these levels are when the fish oil programme is started, usually the greater the fall."

Meanwhile, in Sheffield's Cardiothoracic Unit, Dr Reg Saynor has been investigating the effects of concentrated EPA capsules on angina patients. Studying 92 patients in all, (of which 31 had angina and 46 had had a heart attack) some for up to 2 years. Not only did cholesterol and triglycerides fall, and HDLs rise, but all angina patients were able to stop other medication completely after 9 months on EPA. These results are even more significant when you consider that other diet and lifestyle changes known to reduce heart disease were not changed.

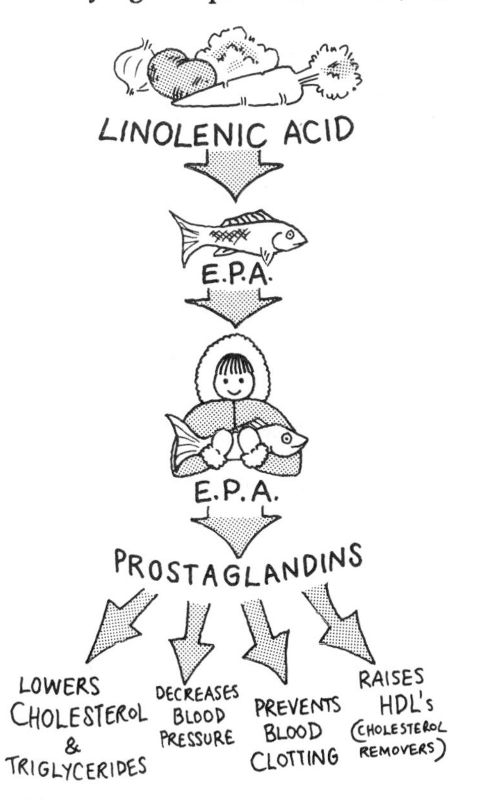

DIAGRAM 4 - The EPA Pathway

But how does EPA work? EPA belongs to a class of fats called Omega 3 fatty acids. The most common type of Omega 3 fatty acid is linolenic acid. This is particularly high in vegetable and seed oils. It is also manufactured by algae which get eaten by small fish, which in turn get eaten by large fish. The fish convert the linolenic acid into EPA. We then turn the EPA into a hormone-like group of substances called *prostaglandins* . One type of prostaglandin, called *thromboxane* stops the blood from clotting, hence lowering the risk of heart disease.

There is little doubt that 'fishitarians', communities eating little meat and lots of fish, plus vegetarian foods, have the lowest heart disease risk. Dr Kromhout and colleagues studied the relationship between fish consumption and mortality from heart disease and concluded "The consumption of as little as one or two fish dishes per week may be of preventive value in relation to heart disease." The best fish to eat are cold water fish like haddock, herring, mackerel, salmon, sardines, anchovies and pilchards. As well as containing EPA they're an excellent source of protein. However the levels of EPA you get from eating fish twice a week is quite alot less than those used in the EPA trials. Taking cod liver oil, although a good source, may not be the answer either. Concentrated capsules of EPA are now available, both in health food shops and on prescription. For those with any risk for heart disease it is wise to supplement your diet with EPA. The minimum level worth taking is 180mg, however up to ten times this amount is far more effective in people with advanced cardiovascular disease.

PREVENTING HIGH BLOOD PRESSURE

Since high blood pressure is a significant risk factor for heart disease a number of drugs have been developed with the aim of reducing blood pressure. The normal procedure for someone with high blood pressure is to advise weight reduction if they are overweight, decrease fat and salt intake. Diuretic drugs are then given which cause the body to excrete excess fluids plus sodium thus reducing blood pressure. Although this effectively reduces blood pressure these drugs do not deal with the root cause of the problem and they promote the excretion of beneficial minerals, including potassium, calcium and magnesium. Other drugs used are not without side-effects. Beta blockers, a class of vasodilator, may cause muscle spasm and depression. There is also some evidence that medication may increase deaths from other causes as illustrated by a study of 12,000 men between the ages of 35 and 57 considered to have a high risk, by the National Heart, Lung and Blood Institute. Half were assigned to a special group who were given medication and advice to reduce cigarettes, fat and cholesterol. The others did nothing. The results showed "no significant difference in the number of deaths from coronary heart disease." However there were 57 per cent more deaths from other causes in the group treated for high blood pressure!

One immediate way to lower your blood pressure is to increase your intake of calcium, magnesium and potassium, and reduce your intake of sodium. Other nutrients that may be helpful are EPA, gamma linolenic acid (usually provided as evening primrose oil) and vitamin B6 which is a mild diuretic.

Reducing your sodium intake, increasing your calcium, magnesium and potassium intake have all been proven to reduce blood pressure. The combined effect of doing all these things at once is likely to reduce a high blood pressure by 10 to 20 per cent if body levels of potassium, calcium and magnesium are low. These results are consistent with studies that have found a low incidence of heart disease in parts of the world where calcium and magnesium intake are high, or in hard water areas, since hard water contains more calcium and magnesium. The best source of potassium is fruit, while calcium is found in dairy produce, vegetables, nuts and seeds. Magnesium is also found in vegetables, nuts and seeds, almonds, sesame and sunflower seeds being particularly good sources. The average British diet provides around 250mg of magnesium a day, compared to the US RDA of 350 to 400mg. A recent survey found that 73 per cent of women in Britain do not get the RDA for calcium.

Magnesium deficiency may have far more serious consequences that just increasing blood pressure. In experiments with dogs decreasing blood levels of magnesium can send arteries into spasm blocking off blood flow. It is known that a number of people who die from heart attacks do not die as a result of arterial occlusion but as a result of coronary artery spasm, or possibly a combination of both. At the moment it is not known how many heart attacks are induced by coronary artery spasm and, if so, to what extent magnesium plays a part. However, there is a strong association between magnesium deficiency and heart disease risk. As well as eating a diet rich in calcium, magnesium and potassium I recommend supplementing around 350mg of calcium and 175mg of magnesium every day.

Other minerals that help to promote a healthy heart are selenium, zinc and manganese. Selenium is a vital component of *glutathione peroxidase* an anti-oxidant enzyme. In 1976 Dr Shamberger first presented evidence showing that people living in areas where selenium levels in the soil are low are more likely to die from heart disease. Since then selenium has been shown to effect blood pressure, prevent atherosclerosis and potentiate the effects of vitamin E. It is commonly deficient in the British diet and subsequently daily supplements of 100mcg are necessary to ensure you receive optimal amounts. Zinc and manganese are involved in another anti-oxidant enzyme called *superoxide dismutase* (SOD for short). In fact, copper is also involved in this enzyme, however an excess of copper interferes with its function and is associated with raised blood pressure. Zinc helps to lower excessive copper levels which are far more common than deficiency due to the widespread use of copper water pipes.

Other toxic elements that raise blood pressure are lead and cadmium. Both of these can be detoxified from the body by increasing intake of zinc, calcium and vitamin C. Car fumes are the main source of lead which reaches us from fall-out onto fruit and vegetables, through our water and the air we breathe. Cadmium is found in cigarettes and is consequently higher in smokers.

CO-ENZYME Q AND HEART DISEASE

Another vital nutrient for the heart rather than the arteries is Co-enzyme Q 10. Co-enzyme Q is a semi-essential nutrient in that it can be made by the body. However recent research suggests that many of us, particularly later in life, do not make enough and can benefit from extra amounts. Co-Q acts as an anti-oxidant and helps all cells to use oxygen more efficiently, which is very important in angina, certain forms of congenital heart disease and for people who have already had a heart attack destroying a proportion of heart muscle.

In a six year study at the University of Texas involving people with congestive heart failure, a condition in which the heart becomes progressively weaker, 75 per cent of those on Co-Q survived three years, compared to 25 per cent on conventional medication. In no less than twenty properly controlled studies published in the last three years Co-Q has repeatedly demonstrated a remarkable ability to improve heart function and has now become the treatment of choice in Japan.

In a combined trial by the University of Austin, Texas and the Centre for Adult Diseases in Osaka, Japan, 52 patients with high blood pressure were treated either with Co-Q or dummy tablets. There was an 11 per cent decrease in blood pressure for those on Co-Q, compared to a 2 per cent decrease for those on dummy tablets. In one study at Hamamatsu University angina patients treated with Co-Q were able to increase their tolerance to exercise and had less frequent angina attacks. After only four weeks on Co-Q other medication had effectively been halved. Although these trials used around 90mg of Co-Q supplementing 30mg a day should have a beneficial effect. Most supplements contain 10mg only.

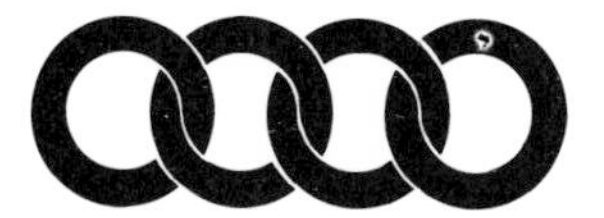

CHAPTER FOUR

HOW TO AVOID HEART DISEASE

BY now you'll realise just how much you can do to prevent cardiovascular disease. You might not be able to make all the changes you'd like to make straight away, but there's a lot you can do without hesitation. Cardiovascular disease isn't something that comes out of the blue. It takes years to develop. Once you've started to correct your less healthful habits and boosted yourself with optimum levels of the right nutrients you can rest assured that your health will improve and your healthy lifespan will be extended. Leading nutritionist Dr Michael Colgan says "Provided you're not already in the grips of a degenerative disease you are likely to get at least a decade of vigorous years, and perhaps a lot more, added to your lifespan, whatever age you are now." Dr Carl Pfeiffer, renowned for his work in treating mental illness with nutrition, is a case in point. At the age of 51 he suffered a massive heart attack. He was given at most, another ten years to live and advised to have a pacemaker fitted. Instead he decided to pursue optimum nutrition both in his life and his work, and made some remarkable breakthroughs in the treatment of mental illness, his speciality. He died of a heart attack at the age of 80, 29 years later, while doing his usual full working day. Dr Linus Pauling, now aged 87, believes that optimum nutrition, plus vitamin C can add 16 to 24 years to the average lifespan. Dr Roger Williams, now aged 95 says "Well rounded nutrition, including generous amounts of vitamin C and E, can contribute materially to extending the healthy lifespan of those who are already middle-aged." The message is clear. The supernutrition approach works and the sooner you start the longer will be your healthy lifespan. Here are some guidelines to help you get started.

THE HEALTHY HEART PLAN

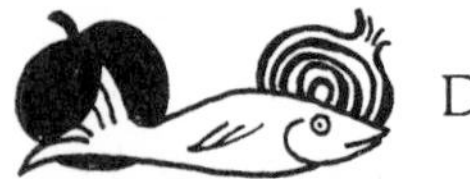

DIET

Avoid Sugar, Salt and Saturated Fat

You don't need sugar and you don't need salt. Once you've developed the taste for sugar it takes some time to break. Start by reducing, or avoiding sugar in hot drinks. If you have sugar on cereal, slice on a banana or some other fruit instead. Start buying sugar-free foods. Nowadays you can get everything from sugar-free biscuits to sugar-free baked beans. They still taste good. When you feel like something sweet eat fresh fruit instead. Set yourself a target every month and gradually wean yourself off sugar. Honey is little better so this is best avoided too. Once you are basically sugar free the odd bit is not going to harm you.

If you are a saltaholic you may well be zinc deficient. A lack of zinc leads to an impaired ability to taste, which can lead to a liking for salty foods. Supplement your diet with 20mg of zinc a day for 2 months then start reducing the amount of salt that you use. After one month without salt, foods that used to taste bland will begin to have some flavour.

It isn't possible, or necessary, to completely avoid saturated fat, but it is wise to reduce it. How? Eat more vegetarian foods and have fish and chicken instead of meat. 75 per cent of the calories in a steak are derived from fat, compared to 40 per cent for chicken and 34 per cent for cod. Don't fry. Grill or bake instead. Have skimmed milk and less cheese. Cottage cheese and edam or gouda are lower in fat. Don't have more than five eggs a week. They're 66 per cent fat. Avoid junk food. A typical fast food burger contains the equivalent of eight pats of butter. The best way the cut down on fat is to fill your diet with low fat foods, including masses of fruit and vegetables. Don't limit the amount you eat of any low fat foods.

Avoid Stimulants

Sugar is a stimulant, and so is chocolate, coffee, tea and cola drinks. Stimulants only give us energy in the short-term by inducing a stress reaction. In this state the body immediately stops repairing itself. The more you use stimulants the faster you age. When your diet and supplement programme is right you'll find you have more than enough energy without needing extra stimulants. The most harmful stimulant is coffee. If you drink coffee do this simple experiment. Avoid it completely for two weeks, then have a strong cup of coffee. This way you'll be able to experience the short-term effect coffee has on your health. Even if you don't experience any short-term effects be sure coffee does you harm in the long run. If you drink tea decrease the amount and strength of the tea you drink, sometimes having herb teas instead. The odd cup of weak tea is not going to harm you if the rest of your diet is good.

Keep Your Alcohol Intake Moderate

Alcohol has many harmful effects, the most of which is that it is addictive. If you haven't had a week without alcohol for a long time try it, see how hooked you've become on a regular drink. From the point of view of cardiovascular disease a glass of wine, beer or spirit a day is unlikely to do you any harm.

Eat for Vitamin and Mineral Vitality

Eat foods rich in the vitamins and minerals that are good for the heart and arteries. For example, have carrots and other red-yellow fruits and vegetables. Citrus fruit, kiwi fruit and green peppers are rich in vitamin C. Wheatgerm, nuts and seeds are rich in vitamin E. Don't leave them lying around for months before you eat them because the oils will go rancid and the vitamin E content will drop. Almonds take longer to go rancid than walnuts or pecans. Brazil nuts are the highest in fat and are best avoided. Sesame and sunflower seeds are less prone to rancidity and, like almonds, are packed with calcium and magnesium. Sesame seeds are a rich source of selenium, as is all seafood. Bananas are a rich source of potassium. A breakfast of low-fat, sugar-free yoghurt, wheatgerm, ground sesame seeds, skimmed milk and a chopped banana gives you protein, vitamin E, calcium, magnesium, selenium, potassium, and many other nutrients. If you'd like some recipes read either The Metabolic Diet or Vitamin Vitality (details on page 47).

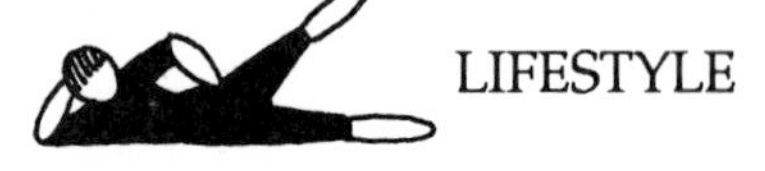

LIFESTYLE

Keep Fit Not Fat

Even 30 minutes a week of aerobic exercise (raising your pulse to 80 per cent of its maximum) is enough to maintain the fitness of your cardiovascular system. More strengthens your heart and arteries. It also helps to boost your metabolic rate and keep you slim. Being overweight puts an extra strain on your heart and arteries. The best forms of exercise are brisk walking, hill walking, jogging, swimming, cycling or aerobics. Find a sport you enjoy and play it once a week. Start doing some regular exercise each week. It might not seem like much to start with but it really makes a difference in the long run.

Avoid Prolonged Stress

Keep cool. Stress raises your blood pressure by causing blood vessels to constrict and the heart to beat faster. Notice your signs of tension (clenched fists, tight shoulders, nail biting, shallow breathing etc.) and observe what circumstances make you react stressfully. Notice how you react. Do you drink more, eat more, become hyperactive, get cross? When you know what causes you stress and how you react you're more than half way there. Then you have two options. Realise that it doesn't serve you to react stressfully in these situations. Or, if you are continually in a situation that causes you stress get out of the situation. You'll handle stress much better if you avoid stimulants.

Stop Smoking

Smoking triggers off cell proliferation, starves healthy cells of oxygen, thickens the blood and raises your blood pressure. Of the deaths caused by smoking twice as many are due to diseases of the heart and arteries than due to lung cancer. The less you smoke the better. But best of all, stop smoking.

Check Your Blood Pressure and Blood Fats

Check your blood pressure and your blood levels of cholesterol, triglycerides and HDLs at least every three years. The older you are the more frequent you should check. Your doctor can do these for you. Make sure you keep a copy of the results so you can compare your levels to those given in this book. When your blood fats and your blood pressure are low you know your risk is minimal.

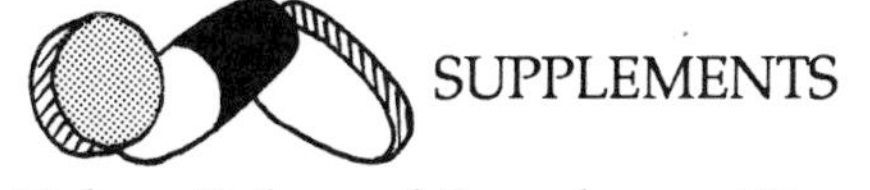

SUPPLEMENTS

Take a Balanced Supplement Programme Every Day

Whatever your opinions about taking supplements the truth is this. The nutrients discussed in this book promote cardiovascular health when taken in the amounts suggested. Even a well balanced diet is unlikely to provide anywhere near these levels. I take supplements every day because I feel better, have seen them literally save people's lives, want to live a long and healthy life, and know that they can only do me good.

Ideal levels vary from person to person and for maximum cardiovascular health I recommend you supplement the levels shown in the chart below, as well as eating as good a diet as you can. I have listed ideal levels for basic prevention and the range for therapeutic use. Therapeutic levels should not be taken without the advice or supervision of your doctor or nutritionist. A directory of qualified nutritionists is available from the Institute for Optimum Nutrition (see page 47 for details).

IDEAL NUTRIENT INTAKE FOR A HEALTHY HEART

NUTRIENT	PREVENTION	THERAPEUTIC RANGE
Vitamin A	**20,000ius**	**20,000 - 35,000ius**
as retinol	**7,500ius**	**7,500-15,000ius**
as beta-carotene	**12,500ius**	**12,500-20,000ius**
Vitamin D	400ius	
Vitamin E	**200ius**	**400-1,000ius**
Vitamin C	**1,000mg**	**2,000-10,000mg**
B1 (Thiamine)	25mg	
B2 (Riboflavin)	25mg	
B3 (Niacin)	**25mg**	**50-250mg**
B5 (Pantothenic acid)	25mg	
B6 (Pyridoxine)	**25mg**	**50-100mg**
B12	10mcg	
Folic acid	100mcg	
Biotin	50mcg	
Calcium	**350mg**	**350-800mg**
Magnesium	**175mg**	**175-500mg**
Zinc	**20mg**	**20-50mg**
Iron	10mg	
Manganese	**2.5mg**	**10-20mg**
Chromium	20mcg	
Selenium	**100mcg**	**100-400mcg**
EPA	**180mg**	**360-3,000mg**

*Most important nutrients are **bold**

The best way to obtain the 'prevention' levels of all these nutrients is to take a special supplement pack containing three tablets and one capsule called **the HH Pack**, made by Health+Plus Ltd (see page 47 for their details). This provides all these levels, together with EPA. When supplementing vitamin E make sure you buy natural d-alpha tocopherol, not mixed tocopherols or dl-alpha tocopherol, which are less potent. When buying mineral supplements check you are getting the elemental value of each mineral. For example, zinc gluconate 20mg actually gives you 2mg of zinc. Reputable manufacturers usually state the elemental value on the label.

Take your supplements with food, unless otherwise stated. Many vitamins help to boost your energy levels so are best taken with breakfast or lunch. Calcium and magnesium have a calming effect and are best taken with dinner, especially if you have difficulty getting to sleep. Most important of all, stick to your supplement programme every day. It can take three months before you notice the beneficial effects. They are worth waiting for.

USEFUL ADDRESSES

HEALTH+PLUS Ltd supply vitamin and mineral supplements, including The HH Pack, by mail order. Ring or write to Health+Plus Ltd, Health+Plus House, 118 Station Road, Chinnor, OXON OX9 4EZ Tel: 0844 52098.

THE INSTITUTE FOR OPTIMUM NUTRITION offers courses and personal consultations with trained nutritionists, including Patrick Holford. A directory of ION-trained nutritionists is available for £1. To receive ION's information pack please ring or write to ION, 5 Jerdan Place, London SW6 1BE Tel: 01 385 7984.

RECOMMENDED READING

The following books will help you dig deeper into nutrition.

Patrick Holford - *Vitamin Vitality* (ION Press) 1985. A thoroughly researched book which establishes why so many people are sub-optimally nourished and how to work out your own vitamin and mineral needs for optimum health.

Patrick Holford - *The Metabolic Diet* (Ebury Press) 1987. This book explains how to boost your metabolic rate and lose weight permanently. As well as explaining the 'mechanics' of weight control, this book is highly practical with a 30 day diet and delicious recipes.

Patrick Holford - *The Family Nutrition Workbook* (Thorsons) 1988. This large format book covers every major topic in nutrition. It is designed as a workbook and condenses all the facts about food you need to know to be healthy and stay healthy. It also teaches you how to analyse your diet and work out your own vitamin needs.

HOW TO BOOST YOUR IMMUNE SYSTEM

by Jennifer Meek

The first in the *Nutrition Connection* series, this book explains how the immune system works and what you can do to make yours healthy. It include the Immune Power Diet, an action plan for immune strength. (£1.99)
ISBN 1-870976-00-2

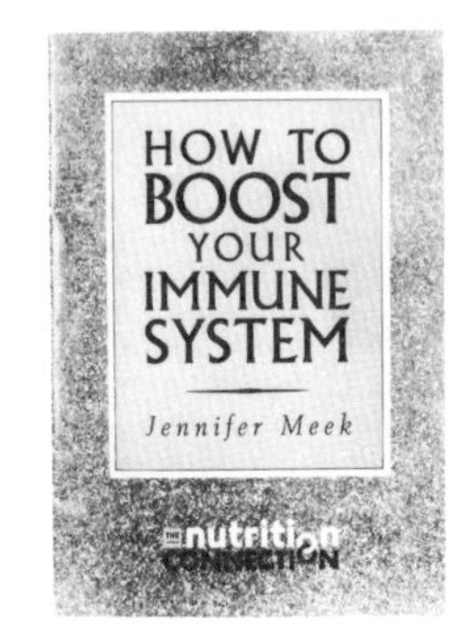

VITAMIN VITALITY

by Patrick Holford

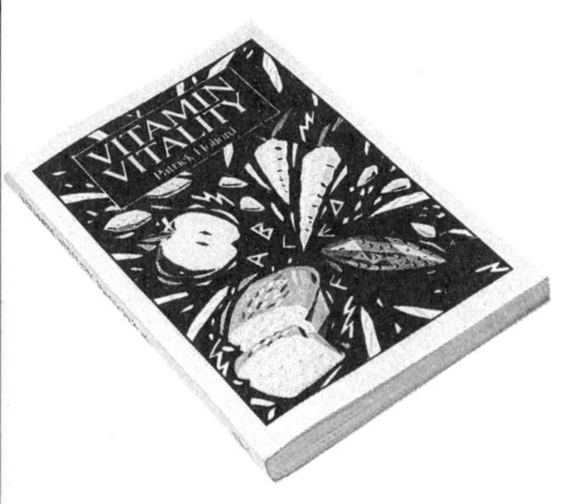

Are you getting all the vitamins you need, even in a well-balanced diet? Patrick Holford presents convincing evidence that 80 per cent of people don't even get the minimum recommended levels.

This topical - at times, controversial - book shows how, with a careful intake of vitamins and minerals, both from your diet and from supplements, you can achieve optimum health and get the very best out of yourself. (£3.95) ISBN 0-00-411979-7

THE ENERGY EQUATION

by Patrick Holford

Energy, or rather lack of it, is the most common sign of ill-health. But what is energy, how do you make it and get more of it? Patrick Holford explains how vital vitamins turn food into energy, and why a newly discovered nutrient, Co-Enzyme Q, is now thought to be the missing link in the energy equation.
ISBN 1 87097 601 0 (£1.99)

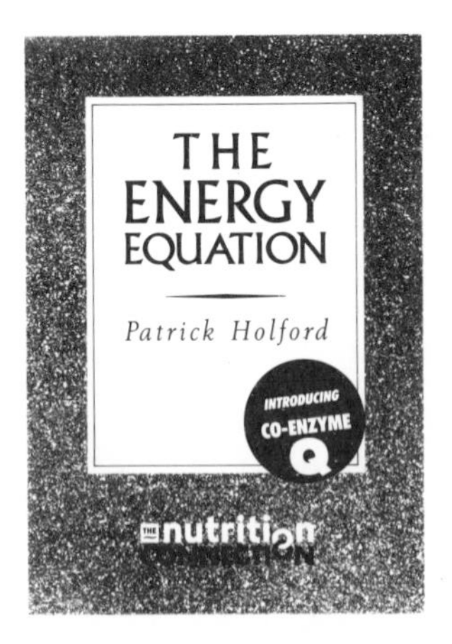

These books can be ordered from any bookshop, or, in case of difficulty, post-free direct from ION Press, 5 Jerdan Place, London SW6 1BE.